The Sirtfood Diet

Lunch

48 Sirtfood Diet Recipes for Beginners - Lose Weight Fast, Burn Fat and Heal Your Body

Lola Ross

Table of Contents

Intruduction

The sirtfood diet has been tested and proven to be the formula that addresses the frustrations of limited weight loss success. Generally, the way to lose weight is through calorie restriction. Since this is not an easy task to accomplish, a dietary plan that focuses on the consumption of sirtuin-activating foods to activate the body's skinny genes was developed. Once this is followed, weight loss becomes achievable. Two celebrities who follow the diet; singer Adele and athlete Pippa Middleton have attributed most of their recent weight loss success to this diet plan. Adele lost more than 40 pounds in a few weeks, and several more, in recent years. Others in- clude models Jodie Kidd and Lorraine Pascale; heavyweight boxer David Haye and Olympic gold medalist Ben Ainslie. Thanks to these celebrities, an increasing number of people are considering a diet that boasts of an initial fat loss of 7 pounds in 7 days, and several other health benefits, including reducing stress, stopping inflammation and boosting metab- olism. What's more, all these are achieved without having to starve oneself or face malnutrition. The Sirtfood diet involves eating certain foods that are packed with sirtuins in order to activate your 'skinny gene' pathway. Until a few years ago, a lot of people didn't know the words, 'skinny gene' existed, let alone its relationship to fat and weight loss and a healthy metabolism. So if you are wondering what this means, you aren't alone. Our skinny genes control our metabolism. They are activated when we eat foods that are packed with sirtuins. Activating your skinny gene is trig- gering your body to burn fat. The main function of the sirtfood diet is to activate or turn on the skinny gene, (SIRT1 gene) so as to prevent fat storage and increase the body's fat burning metabolism.

What is The Sirtfood Diet?

Launched originally in 2016, the Sirtfood diet remains a hot topic and involves followers adopting a diet rich in 'sirtfoods'. According to the diet's founders, these special foods work by activating specific proteins in the body called sirtuins. Sirtuins are believed to protect cells in the body from dying when they are under stress and are thought to regulate inflammation, metabolism, and the aging process. It's thought that sirtuins influence the body's ability to burn fat and boost metabolism, resulting in a seven-pound weight loss a week while maintaining muscle. However, some experts believe this is unlikely to be solely fat loss, but will instead reflect changes in glycogen stores from skeletal muscle and the liver.

So What Are These Magical 'Sirtfoods'?   The Twenty Most Common Include:

❖ kale
❖ red wine
❖ strawberries
❖ onions

- ❖ soy
- ❖ parsley
- ❖ extra virgin olive oil
- ❖ dark chocolate (85% cocoa)
- ❖ matcha green tea
- ❖ buckwheat
- ❖ turmeric
- ❖ walnuts
- ❖ arugula (rocket)
- ❖ bird's eye chili
- ❖ lovage
- ❖ Medjool dates
- ❖ red chicory
- ❖ blueberries
- ❖ capers
- ❖ coffee

The diet is divided into two phases; the initial phase lasts one week and involves restricting calories to 1000kcal for three days, consuming three sirtfood green juices, and one meal rich in sirtfoods each day. The juices include kale, celery, rocket, parsley, green tea, and lemon. Meals include turkey escalope with sage, capers and parsley, chicken and kale curry, and prawn stir-fry with buckwheat noodles. From days four to seven, energy intakes are increased to 1500kcal comprising of two sirtfood green juices and two sirtfood-rich meals a day. Although the diet promotes healthy foods, it's restrictive in both your food choices and daily calories, especially during the initial stages. It also involves drinking juice, with the amounts suggested during phase one exceeding the current daily guidelines.

The second phase is known as the maintenance phase which lasts 14 days where steady weight loss occurs. The authors believe it's a sustainable and realistic way to lose weight. However, focusing on weight loss is not what the diet is all about – it's designed to be about eating the best foods nature has to offer. Long term they recommend eating three balanced sirtfood rich meals a day along with one sirtfood green juice.

Dietitian Emer Delaney Says:

'At first glance, this is not a diet I would advise for my clients. Aiming to have 1000kcal for three consecutive days is extremely difficult and I believe the majority of people would be unable to achieve it. Looking at the list of foods, you can see they are the sort of items that often appear on a 'healthy food list', however it would be better to encourage these as part of a healthy balanced diet. Having a glass of red wine or a small amount of chocolate occasionally won't do us any harm – I wouldn't recommend them daily. We should also be eating a mixture of different fruits and vegetables and not just those on the list.

'In terms of weight loss and boosting metabolism, people may have experienced a seven-pound weight loss on the scales, but in my experience, this will be fluid. Burning and losing fat takes time so it is extremely unlikely this weight loss is a loss of fat. I would be very cautious of any diet that recommends fast and sudden weight loss as this simply isn't achievable and will more than likely be a loss of fluid. As soon as people return to their regular eating habits, they will regain the weight. Slow and steady weight loss is the key and for this, we need to restrict calories and increase our activity levels. Eating balanced regular meals made up of low GI foods, lean protein, fruit, and vegetables, and keeping well hydrated is the safest way to lose weight.'

The Health Benefits

There is growing evidence that sirtuin activators may have a wide range of health benefits as well as building muscle and suppressing appetite. These include improving memory, helping the body better control blood sugar levels, and cleaning up the damage from free radical molecules that can accumulate in cells and lead to cancer and other diseases.

'Substantial observational evidence exists for the beneficial effects of the intake of food and drinks rich in sirtuin activators in decreasing risks of chronic disease,' said Professor Frank Hu, an expert in nutrition and epidemiology at Harvard University in a recent article in the journal Advances In Nutrition. A Sirt food diet is particularly suitable as an anti-aging regime.

Although sirtuin activators are found all through the plant kingdom, only certain fruits and vegetables have large enough amounts to counting as Sirt foods. Examples include green tea, cocoa powder, the Indian spice turmeric, kale, onions, and parsley. Many of the fruit and vegetables on display in supermarkets, such as tomatoes, avocados, bananas, lettuce, kiwis, carrots, and cucumber, are rather low in sirtuin activators. This doesn't mean that they aren't worth eating, though, as they provide lots of other benefits.

A remarkable finding of one Sirt food diet trial is that participants lost substantial weight without losing muscle. It was common for participants to gain muscle, leading to a more defined and toned look. That's the beauty of sirtfoods; they activate fat burning but also promote muscle growth, maintenance, and repair. This is in complete contrast to other diets where weight loss typically comes from both fat and muscle, with the loss of muscle slowing down metabolism and making weight regain more likely.

In terms of weight loss and boosting metabolism, people may have experienced a seven-pound weight loss on the scales, but in my experience, this will be fluid. Burning and losing fat takes time so it is extremely unlikely this weight loss is a loss of fat. I would be very cautious of any diet that recommends fast and sudden weight loss as this simply isn't achievable and will more than likely be a loss of fluid. As soon as people return to their regular eating habits, they will regain the weight. Slow and steady weight loss is the key and for this, we need to restrict calories and increase our activity levels. Eating balanced regular meals made up of low GI foods, lean protein, fruit, and vegetables, and keeping well hydrated is the safest way to lose weight.'

1. Hearty Chicken And Bean Casserole

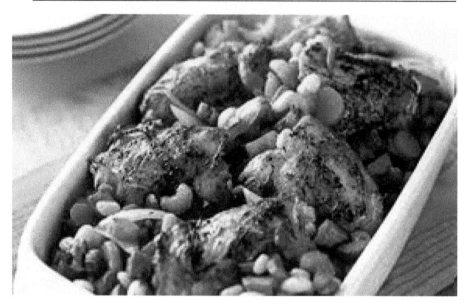

Prep Time: 30 minutes Cook Time: 1 hr.22 minutes Servings: 6

Ingredients

8 oz. (1-1/4 cups) dried Great Northern beans

1 tablespoon olive oil

6 chicken thighs (approx. 2-1/4 pounds total), skinned

1 medium red onion, cut thinly into wedges

2 medium carrots, sliced thinly 1 stalk celery, sliced 2 garlic cloves, minced

1 14.5 oz. can diced tomatoes, no-salt-added, un-drained

6 oz. cooked smoked sausage, cut into pieces

½ teaspoon of crushed dried thyme

¼ teaspoon salt

¼ teaspoon cayenne pepper

Directions

1. Rinse the beans by placing in a large saucepan. Add 4 cups of cold water and bring to a boil. Lower heat, uncover and simmer for 2 minutes. Remove. Cover and set aside for 1 hour. Drain and rinse beans. 2. Preheat oven to 350°F. Heat oil in a large skillet over medium-high. Add the chicken; lower heat and cook 10 minutes until brown on both sides. Remove chick- en. Drain the drippings from skillet, reserving just 1 tablespoon. 3. Add the carrots, onion, the celery, and the garlic to the skillet of drippings. Cover and cook about 10 minutes. Add the drained beans, the tomatoes, stir and then add the sausage, the thyme, salt, and, cayenne pepper. Let it boil. 4. Remove to a baking dish. Place the chicken thighs on top and bake for about 25 minutes, without covering.

Nutrition Facts: Per Serving; Calories 347; Fat 10g; Carbohyd rates 32g; Protein 33g; Fiber 10g; Sodium: 481mg; Cholesterol: 98mg

2. Sautéed Green Beans And Red Onion

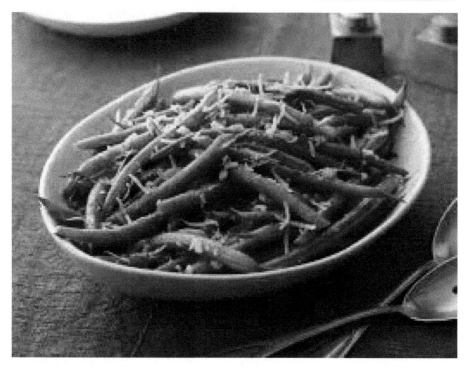

Prep Time: 10 minutes Cook Time: 20 minutes Servings: 4

Ingredients

1 cup of water

2 tablespoons extra virgin olive oil

1 teaspoon kosher salt

1/4teaspoon ground pepper 1lb. green beans

1 medium red onion, cut into wedges

2 teaspoons of balsamic vinegar

Directions

1. Add the water, olive oil, salt, and pepper to a skillet and a simmer over medi- um heat.

2. Add the trimmed and halved green beans and the red onion.

3. Cook, covered for 10 minutes.

4. Uncover and keep cooking and stirring for about 6-7 more minutes until the water has evaporated. Add the vinegar, stir and serve.

Nutrition Facts:

Per Serving; Calories 108.5; Fat 7g; Carbohydrates 11g; Protein 2.4g; Fiber 3.6g;Sodium 591.8 mg; Cholesterol 0 mg

3. Roasted Salmon Tomatoes With Horseradish

Prep Time: 15 minutes Cook Time: 22 minutes Servings: 4

Ingredients

4 (6-oz.) salmon fillets

3/4 teaspoon of kosher salt, divided

1/2 teaspoon black pepper

1/4 cup fresh horseradish, grated (from 1 8-oz. horseradish root)

1 tablespoon shallot, finely chopped

2 tablespoons capers

4 tablespoons + 1 teaspoon of extra virgin olive oil, divided 6 cups of grape tomatoes

1 cup (1 oz.) arugula

3 tablespoons roasted pistachios, unsalted, chopped 2 teaspoons fresh thyme, chopped

Directions

1. Preheat oven to 450°F.

2. Line baking pan with parchment paper and place the salmon on it, with the

skin side facing down in the centre of the baking sheet/pan. Sprinkle with 1/2 tea- spoon salt and the pepper.

3. In a bowl, combine the horseradish, shallot, drained and chopped capers and 2 tablespoons of oil in a bowl.

4. Spread mixture over salmon, pressing lightly. Place the tomatoes around the salmon, and drizzle it with 2 tablespoons of oil.

5. Roast 20 minutes or thereabouts, and then broil for 2 minutes, or until the tomatoes and toppings are brown.

6. Combine the arugula and the reserved oil together. Sprinkle the tomatoes with the arugula. Add the thyme and salt. Serve!

Nutrition Facts:

Per Serving; Calories 464 ; Fat 27g; Carbohydrates 15g; Protein 40g; Fiber 5g;Sodium: 673mg; Cholesterol: 90mg

4. Autumn Stuffed Enchiladas

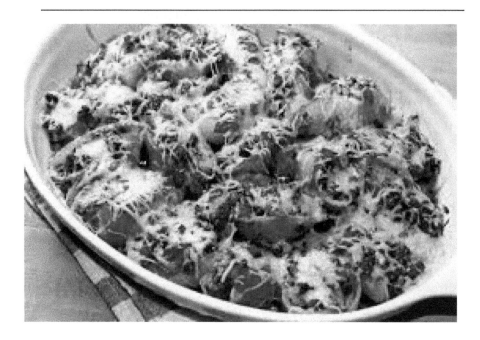

Total time:1 hour

Servings: 4

Ingredients:

1 lemon, juiced

1 cup cashews

½ oz. parsley

1 oz. roasted pumpkin seeds

8 corn tortillas

2 cups Butternut squash

1 cup salsa

1 can black beans

2 tbsp. olive oil

¼ tbsp. cayenne pepper

1 tsp. chili flakes

1 tsp. cumin

3 cloves garlic

1 jalapeno

1 red onion

1 cup Brussels sprouts

Directions:

1. Soak the cashews in boiling water and set aside.
2. Cut the squash in half, and after scooping out the seeds, lightly rub olive oil.
3. Sprinkle with a little salt and pepper before putting on a baking sheet face down. Cook for about forty-five minutes at 400°F until it is cooked.
4. Heat one tbsp. olive oil in a pan on medium heat and put chopped onion in, stirring until soft. Finely dice the jalapeno and garlic and finely slice the Brussel
5. sprouts. Add these three things to the frypan and cook until the Brussels begin to wilt through.
6. Strain and rinse the black beans, then add them to the frypan and mix well.
7. When the squash is cooked and cool enough to handle, scrape out the soft insides away from the skin and put in

a big bowl along with the Brussels mixture. Mix well again with salt and pepper to taste.

8. Put the tortillas in the oven to soften up (don't let them get crispy)

9. Spoon the squash mixture into the middle of the soft tortillas. Carefully roll them up to make little open-ended wraps, and then put in on a baking tray with the open ends down to stop them from unrolling.

10. Do this for all twelve tortillas, then pour the rest of the salsa on top and spread to coat evenly.

11. Change the temperature of the oven to 350°F and bake for 30 minutes.

12. While these cooks put the drained, soaked cashews into a blender with one and a half cups cold water, lemon juice, and a quarter tsp. salt.

13. Blend until smooth, adding water if it becomes too thick; this is your sour cream.

14. When enchiladas are done, leave to cool while you chop parsley.

15. Then drizzle the sour cream generously over the dish and top with parsley and pumpkin seeds.

Nutrition Facts: Calories: 333kcal; Fat: 11g Carbohydrate: 36g; Protein: 14g;

5. Asian Chicken Drumsticks

Total time: 36 Minutes Servings:2

Ingredients:

6 chicken drumsticks

1/4 cup rice vinegar

3 tbsp. agave syrup

2 tbsp. chicken stock

1 tbsp. lower-sodium soy sauce

1 tbsp. sesame oil

1 tbsp. tomato paste

1 garlic clove, crushed

2 tbsp. walnuts, chopped

½ tsp. turmeric

Directions:

1. Put the chicken in a single layer in the oven and cook at 400°F until the skin is crispy (around 25to 28 minutes), turning drumsticks over partway through cooking.

2. In the meantime, mix vinegar, stock, agave, soy sauce, oil, tomato paste, and garlic in a skillet. Bring to a boil over medium-high.

3. Cook for about 6 minutes until thickened. Put the drumsticks and sauce in a bowl and toss to cover. Sprinkle with walnuts.

Nutrition Facts: Calories 488 Fat 30g Protein 25g Fiber 1g Sugars 26g

6. Zucchini Cream

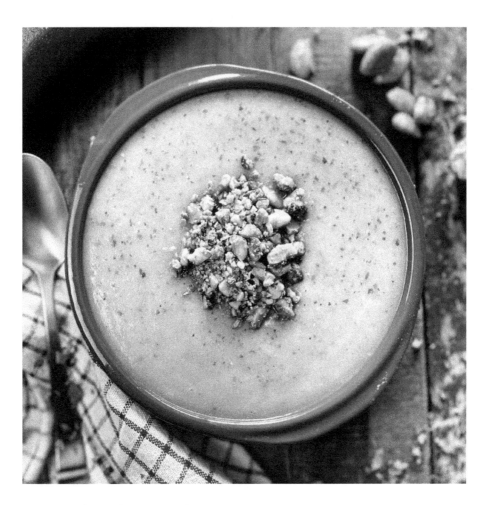

Preparation Time: 10 minutes

Cooking Time: 25 minutes

Servings: 8

Ingredients:

4 cups vegetable stock

2 tablespoons olive oil

2 sweet potatoes, peeled and cubed

8 zucchinis, chopped

2 onions, peeled and chopped

1 cup coconut milk

A pinch of salt and black pepper

1 teaspoon dried rosemary

4 tablespoons fresh dill, chopped

½ teaspoon fresh basil, chopped

Directions:

1. Heat a pot with the oil over medium heat, add the onion, stir, and cook for 2 minutes.
2. Add the zucchinis and the rest of the ingredients except the milk and dill, stir and simmer for 20 minutes.
3. Add the milk and dill, puree the soup using an immersion blender, stir, ladle into soup bowls and serve.

Nutrition: Calories: 324 Carbohydrates: 10g Protein: 14.8g Fat: 3g Sugar: 1.8g Sodium: 585mg Fiber: 0.4g

7. Vinaigrette

Preparation Time: 5 minutes

Cooking Time: 0 minutes

Servings: 1 cup

Ingredients:

4 teaspoons Mustard yellow

4 tablespoon White wine vinegar

1 teaspoon Honey

165 ml Olive oil

Directions:

1. Whisk the mustard, vinegar, and honey in a bowl with a whisk until they are well mixed.
2. Add the olive oil in small amounts while whisking with a whisk until the vinaigrette is thick.
3. Season with salt and pepper.

Nutrition: Calories: 45 Cal Fat: 0.67 g Carbs: 7.18 g Protein: 0.79 g Fiber: 0.8 g

8. Spicy Steak Rolls

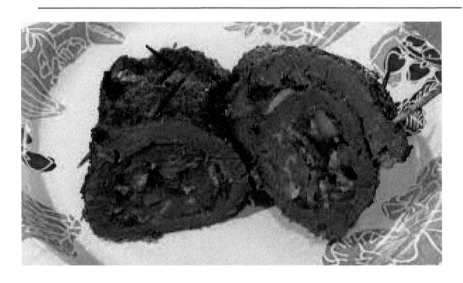

Preparation Time: 20 minutes

Cooking Time: 1 hour 15 minutes

Servings: 4

Ingredients:

    10 slices bacon, chopped

    1 (8 oz.) package fresh mushrooms, chopped

    1 green bell pepper, chopped

    1/2 small onion, chopped

    1 clove garlic, minced, or to taste

    4 beef round steaks

    1/2 cup Montreal steak seasoning

    Toothpicks

Directions:

1. In a large skillet, sauté bacon for about 10 minutes over medium-high heat until evenly browned.
2. Add garlic, onion, green bell pepper, and mushrooms; sauté for about 10 minutes until mushrooms are tender. Put off the heat.
3. Turn an outdoor grill to medium-high and lightly grease the grate.
4. On a flat work surface, position a round steak between 2 pieces of plastic wrap.
5. Use a meat tenderizer to flatten the steak. Do the same with the remaining steaks.

6. Place Montreal steak seasoning into a shallow bowl. Dip 1 side of each steak into the seasoning and place on a cutting board, seasoning-side down.
7. Spread some of the mushroom mixture over the center of each steak. Roll up and secure with toothpicks.
8. Grill the rolled steaks for about 35 minutes on the preheated grill, turning once in a while, until they reach your desired doneness.
9. Take off the toothpicks before serving.

Nutrition: Calories: 163 Carbohydrates: 45.6 g Protein: 3 g Fat: 0.6g

Sugar: 1g Sodium: 87mg Fiber: 0.7 g

9. Spicy Ras-El-Hanout Dressing

Preparation Time: 10 minutes

Cooking Time: 5 minutes

Servings: 1 cup

Ingredients:

125 ml olive oil

1 piece lemon (the juice)

2 teaspoons honey

1 ½ teaspoon Ras el Hanout

½ pieces red pepper

Directions:

1. Remove the seeds from the chili pepper.
2. Chop the chili pepper as finely as possible.
3. Place the pepper in a bowl with lemon juice, honey, and Ras-El-Hanout and whisk with a whisk.
4. Then add the olive oil drop by drop while continuing to whisk.

Nutrition: Calories: 81 Cal Fat: 0.86 g Carbs: 20.02 g Protein: 1.32 g Fiber: 0.9 g

10. Baked Potatoes With Spicy Chickpea Stew

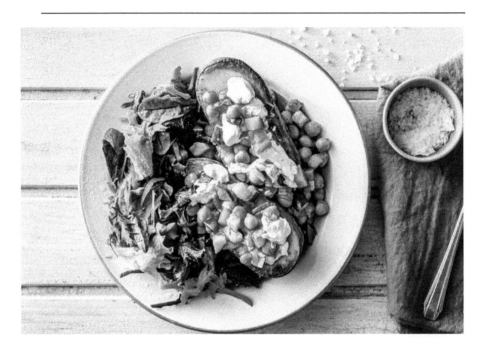

Total time: 70 minutes

Servings: 4

Ingredients:

4 baking potatoes, pricked around

2 tbsp. olive oil

2 red onions, finely chopped

4 tsp. garlic, crushed or grated

1-inch ginger, grated

1/2 tsp. chili flakes

2 tbsp. cumin seeds

2 tbsp. turmeric

2 tins chopped tomatoes

2 tbsp. cocoa powder, unsweetened

2 tins chickpeas – do not drain

2 yellow peppers, chopped

Directions:

1. Preheat the oven to 400°F, and start preparing all ingredients. When the oven is ready, put in baking potatoes and cook for 50 minutes to 1 hour until they are done.
2. While potatoes are cooking, put olive oil and sliced red onion into a wide saucepan and cook lightly, using the lid, for 5 minutes until the onions are tender but not brown.
3. Remove the lid and add ginger, garlic, cumin, and cook for another minute on very low heat. Then add the turmeric and a tiny dab of water and cook for a few more minutes until it becomes thicker, and the consistency is ok.
4. Then add tomatoes, cocoa powder, peppers, chickpeas with their water and salt. Bring to the boil, and then simmer on a very low heat for 45 to 50 minutes until it's thick.

5. Finally, stir in the 2 tbsp. of parsley, some pepper and salt if you desire, and serve the stew with the potatoes.

Nutrition Facts: Calories: 520 Fat: 8g Carbohydrate: 91g Protein: 32g

11. Chicken Kofte with Zucchini

Total time: 52 Minutes

Servings:4

Ingredients:

1/2 cup low-fat Greek yogurt

2 tbsp. black olives, pitted and chopped

1 handful parsley, chopped

1/4 cup breadcrumbs

1/2 red onion, cubed

1 tbsp. ground cumin

1/8 tbsp. chili flakes

1-lb. ground chicken

4 tbsp. olive oil

4 zucchini, sliced

Directions:

1. Mix yogurt, black olives, parsley, breadcrumbs, onion, 1/2 tbsp. salt, and 1/4 tbsp. pepper in a bowl, mixing with a whisk. Add chicken; blend in with hands.
2. Shape chicken mixture into 8 patties. Heat 2 tbsp. olive oil in a skillet over medium heat. Add patties; cook 4 minutes on each side or until done.

3. While kofte cooks, cook zucchini on a skillet. Brush them with 2 tbsp oil and season with the remaining pepper.
4. Cook on high heat for 5 minutes, then season with salt. Serve 2 kofte per person with zucchini on the side.

Nutrition Facts: Calories 301 Fat 16.9g Protein 24g Carbohydrate

15g

12. Beef & Buckwheat Noodles With Mushrooms

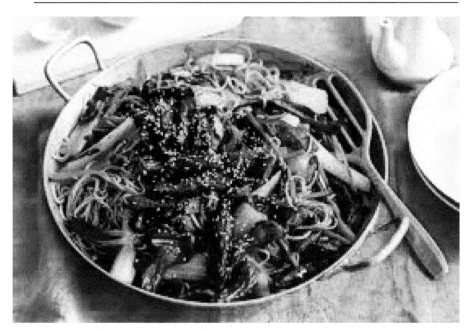

Time: 30 minutes Cook Time: 6 hours 30minutes Servings: 6

Ingredients

1 boneless beef roast (2 lb.), trimmed

1 tablespoon steak seasoning

½ teaspoon of salt

½ teaspoon black pepper

2 tablespoons of extra virgin olive oil

½ cup of red wine

1 onion, diced

1 tablespoon of garlic, minced

3 sprigs thyme

1 bay leaf

4 cups reduced- sodium beef broth

1 tablespoon of Worcestershire sauce

12 ounce buckwheat noodles

2 tablespoons of butter, unsalted

8 oz. button mushrooms, sliced

½ cup of heavy cream

Fresh chives, chopped

Directions

1. Combine steak seasoning and the salt and pepper in a bowl and rub all over the roast.

2. Add the oil to pan and once hot, add the seasoned roast then brown all over for 10 minutes on both sides. Remove to a slow cooker.

3. Add wine to pan to deglaze, and then add to the roast in the slow cooker. Top with the onions, thyme and the bay leaf. Place lid on and cook for 5 hours on high or 8 hours on low.

4. Remove to a cutting board, cut largely, trimming away excess fat, if any, and discarding the bay leaf and thyme springs. Cover with foil.

5. Add the broth, Worcestershire, and noodles to a slow cooker. Let it cook, covered for 1 hour on high. Add the mushrooms and cook for about 10 minutes until liquid evaporates.

Nutrition Facts:

Per Serving; Calories 565 ; Fat 25g; Carbohydrates 36g; Protein 43g; Fiber 1g;Sodium: 711mg; Cholesterol: 197mg

13. Overnight Lemony Limed Brined Pork Ribs

Prep Time: 45minutes Cook Time: 1 hour Servings: 4

Ingredients

1 red onion

3 garlic cloves

2 bay leaves

1/4 cup of kosher salt

1 tablespoon celery seeds

1/2 cup brown sugar 1 tablespoon whole peppercorns 2 cups chicken broth, low sodium

2 lemons

2 limes

5 sprigs sage

2 tablespoons of Dijon mustard

1/2 cup of olive oil

1 teaspoon apple cider vinegar

1 tablespoon honey 1(5 lb.) pork ribs

Directions

1. Cut off the ends of the red onion, peel and cut in half. Cut the pork ribs into 4 portions.

2. Add the red onion to a sauce pot, along with the garlic cloves, bay leaf, the salt, celery seeds, brown sugar, peppercorns and the low sodium chicken broth.

3. Simmer the brine on medium heat until the salt and sugar are fully dissolved. Transfer to a large bowl.

4. Pour in 2 cups of cold water to the brine, and then add 5 ice cubes, lime and lemon juice with their pulp and sage springs. Let it cool and then add the ribs. Leave overnight to soak.

5. Add together the Dijon, vinegar, honey and olive oil to a small bowl. Cover and let it rest overnight as well.

6. When ready to cook, turn grill on and preheat for 15 minutes on medium temperature. Clean the grill carefully with a brush and lower temperature to low. Remove ribs from brine, place on the grill, close and cook for 20 minutes.

7. Open grill, season the ribs with ¼ of the Dijon dressing. Turn the other side and brush with ¼ of the dressing also. Close and cook 20 more minutes.

8. Take off ribs from grill and brush with the rest of the dressing. Serve!

Nutrition Facts:
Per Serving; Calories 472; Fat 44g; Carbohydrates 4g; Protein

14. Chicken Salad With Lemon, Zucchini And Nuts

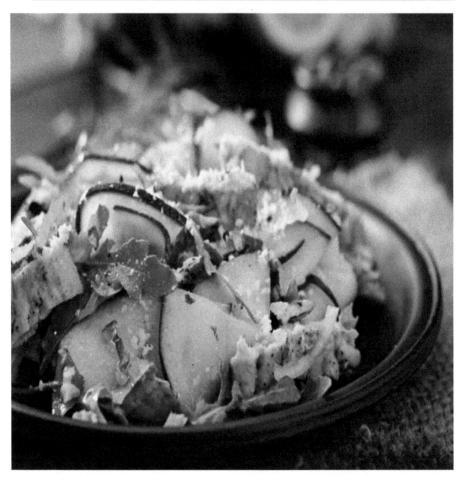

Prep Time: 2 hours 35minutes Cook Time: 10 minutes Servings: 4

Ingredients

1/3 cup of dried currants

1/4 cup extra-virgin olive oil + plus

2 tablespoons

1 clove garlic, sliced thinly

1/8 teaspoon ground cumin Zest of

1 lemon Juice of 2 lemons Kosher salt and fresh ground pepper

3 medium zucchini (2 lb.), cut into sticks

1 large shallot, minced 3 tablespoons pine nuts

1 1/2 lb. skinless, boneless chicken breast halves

2 cups baby arugula leaves

Directions

1. Place the currants in a small bowl. Add hot water and let it stand for 10 min- utes to soften. Drain afterwards.

2. Add together the 2 tablespoons of the oil along with the garlic, cumin, finely grated lemon zest, 1/2 of the lemon juice, ¼ teaspoon of pepper and ½ teaspoon of salt.

3. Add the zucchini sticks and the drained currants and toss. Let it rest for 2 hours, but stir occasionally.

4. Add together the minced shallot and 2 tablespoon oil in a large and shallow dish. Add the remaining lemon juice as well. Add the chicken breast halves and flip to coat. Cover and chill for 1 hour in the refrigerator, flipping occasionally.

5. Toast the pine nuts in a skillet, with some tossing for about 2 minutes and remove to cool in a plate once golden brown.

6. Take out the chicken breast from the marinade and scrape off the shallot. Cut diagonally to 11/2 inch thick slices and then sprinkle with salt and pepper.

7. Heat the remaining oil to a large skillet and once hot, add the chicken and cook for about 8 minutes, flipping a few times until cooked through.

8. Let the chicken slices cool for a while and then serve with the vegetables and currant and toasted pine nuts.

Nutrition Facts:

Per Serving; Calories 544; Fat 24g; Carbohydrates 24g; Protein 5 8g; Fiber 4g; Sodium: 515mg; Cholesterol: 146mg

15.   Sesame Chicken Salad

Prep Time: 15minutes Cook Time: 10 minutes Servings: 6

Ingredients

2 whole boneless, skinless chicken breasts Kosher salt & pepper

2/3 cup extra virgin olive oil

1/4 cup rice wine vinegar

1/4 cup reduced sodium soy sauce 2 tablespoons of minced fresh ginger

2 cloves garlic, minced

2 tablespoons of brown sugar

1 teaspoon toasted sesame oil Pinch crushed red pepper flakes 1 package (10 oz.) mixed greens

1/2 whole red onion, sliced thinly

1 cup of red grape tomatoes, halved

1 can mandarin oranges, drained

1 tablespoon of sesame seeds

1 tablespoon of black sesame seeds

Directions

1. In a blender, add together the olive oil, vinegar, soy sauce, ginger, garlic, brown sugar, sesame oil, and crushed red pepper flakes. Blend thoroughly. Taste and adjust accordingly, adding more or less ingredient as desired.

2. Sprinkle both sides of the chicken with salt and pepper. Grill in a pan or brown in a skillet with oil for 10 minutes. Remove, cool and cut into cubes.

3. Transfer cubed chicken to a bowl. Pour 1/3 of the dressing over, tossing to coat. Let it rest for 2-3 minutes and then add the sesame seeds to it. Toss to coat with the chicken.

4. Assemble salad by placing the greens, sliced onion and the tomatoes in a bowl. Add 1/2 of the dressing or more as desired. Toss and place the chicken and oranges over the salad greens. Serve!

Nutrition Facts:

Per Serving; Calories 704; Fat 35g; Carbohydrates 16g; Protein 8 3g; Fiber 1g; Sodium: 762mg; Cholesterol: 275mg

16.   Baked Salmon With Lemon Caper Butter

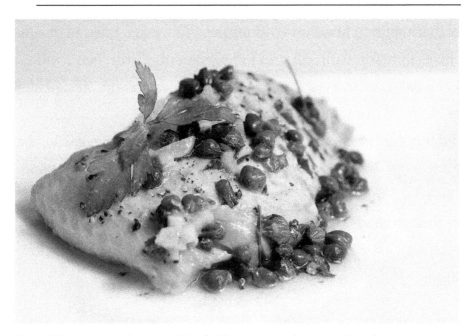

Prep Time: 15 minutes Cook Time: 12 minutes Servings: 2

Ingredients

2 (4-5 oz.) salmon fillets Salt and pepper, to taste

4 lemon slices Lemon Caper Butter

3 tablespoons butter, unsalted

2 cloves garlic, minced

2 tablespoons capers, drained and rinsed Juice of 1/2 of a lemon

1/2 teaspoon lemon zest Kosher

salt and fresh pepper

Directions

1. Preheat oven to 450°F.

2. Place salmon fillets on an aluminum-foiled and greased baking sheet. Sprinkle with salt and pepper and top with lemon slices. Let it bake 10 minutes. Remove from oven, cover with the foil and let it rest for 10 minutes.

3. Melt the unsalted butter in a pan and then add the garlic, the rinsed and drained capers as well as the juice and zest of lemon. Cook for 2 minutes and then add the salt and pepper to season.

4. Remove and discard lemon slices. Remove skin of fillet gently with a spatula. Place fillet on a plate, top with lemon caper butter. Enjoy!

Nutrition Facts:

Per Serving; Calories 323 ; Fat 26.2g; Carbohydrates 2.9g; Pro- t ein 28.3g; Fiber 0.8g;Sodium: 442mg; Cholesterol: 108mg

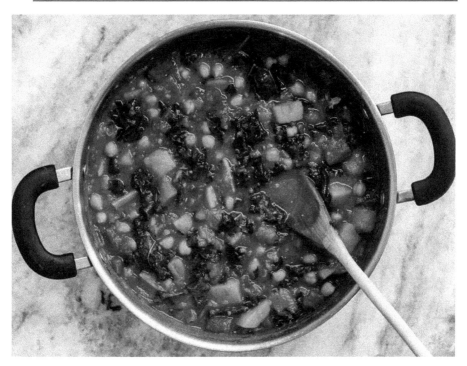

Prep Time: 10 minutes Cook Time: 1 hour Servings: 1.3 cups

Ingredients

2 tablespoons of extra-virgin olive oil

1 teaspoon fresh ginger, grated

2 cloves garlic, minced

1 red onion, diced finely

1 tablespoon turmeric

1 tablespoon of smoked paprika

1 teaspoon chili flakes

1 15oz. can of fire roasted diced tomatoes 2 russet potatoes (about 2 lbs. total), peeled & cubed

4 cups vegetable broth

1 15oz. can chickpeas

1/4 lb. fresh kale, chopped

Directions

1. In a large pot, sauté the onion, the garlic and ginger in olive oil until tender.

2. Add the turmeric, the smoked paprika, and chilli flakes, Cook and stir for 2 minutes.

3. Add the cubed potatoes, diced tomatoes, inclusive of their juices, and then add the drained chickpeas. Pour in the broth and stir to combine all. Cover, raise heat to medium high, and bring to a boil.

4. Lower heat and let the soup simmer, covered for 45 minutes, but with occasional stirring.

5. Mash the potatoes in the pot. Stir in the chopped kale until wilted. Adjust seasoning. Serve hot with crackers or crusty bread.

Nutrition Facts:

Per Serving; Calories 300.78; Fat 7.12g; Carbohydrates 53.15g; Protein 9.92g; Fiber 9.45g; Sodium: 884mg;

18. Spicy Garlic Shrimp with Lemon & Asparagus

Prep Time: 25minutes Cook Time: 10minutes Servings: 4

Ingredients

1 lb. shrimp

3/4 teaspoon kosher salt Freshly ground black pepper 1 lemon 6 tablespoons of extra-virgin olive oil

4 cloves garlic, sliced thinly

3/4 lb. asparagus, (2 cups)

1/4 teaspoon of crushed red pepper flakes

2/3 cup low-sodium chicken broth

1/2 teaspoon of cornstarch

Directions

1. Peel the shrimp, devein, rinse and pat dry with a paper towel. Season the shrimp with black pepper and

1/4 teaspoon salt. Set aside.

2. Shave the zest gently from the lemon in strips. Use a peeler for this. Squeeze the lemon to extract 1 tablespoon of juice.

3. Snap off the bottoms of the asparagus, cut in half and then cut into 2 inches long. This should get you 2 cups asparagus.

4. Add 2 tablespoons of oil to a large skillet. Cook the shrimp in hot oil for 2 minutes. Flip and cook another minute. Remove the slightly cooked shrimp to a plate.

5. Lower heat. Add the remaining oil. Cook the garlic in the oil for 30 seconds. Add the prepared asparagus, the zest of lemon and the red pepper flakes. Add ½ teaspoon of salt. Toss everything together and cook for 3 minutes. Add the broth, place lid on, but leave it ajar. Cook for a minute or two until the asparagus is soft- ened.

6. Combine the cornstarch with a tablespoon of water. Add to the asparagus mixture, stirring well. Let it boil; add the shrimp, lower heat. Cook and toss for 1-2 minutes.

7. Once shrimp is pink, add the lemon juice, stir and then add the salt and pep- per as well as extra lemon juice. Serve!

Nutrition Facts:

Per Serving; Calories 380; Fat 58g; Carbohydrates 50g; Protein 39g; Fiber 18g; Sodium: 735mg; Cholesterol 76mg

19.   Kale Salad with Mocorran-styled Spiced Tofu & Chickpeas

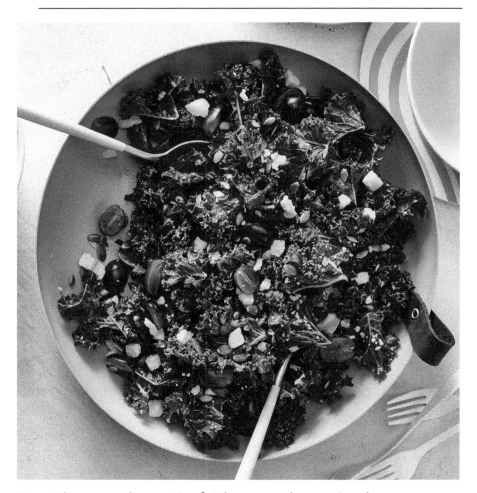

Prep Time: 30minutes Cook Time: 20minutes Servings: 4

Ingredients

3½ teaspoons of ground cumin

3½ teaspoons of paprika

2 teaspoons of garlic powder

¾ teaspoon of salt

1 teaspoon of fresh ground pepper

5 tablespoons of lemon juice, divided

4 tablespoons of extra-virgin olive oil, divided

1 14-oz. package water-packed tofu, extra-firm, drained

1 15-ounce can chickpeas, rinsed

14 cups kale, torn

1/2 English cucumber, cut in two & sliced

1 medium bell pepper, cut into strips

Directions

1. Preheat your oven to 450°F

2. In a large bowl, add together cumin, paprika, garlic powder, salt and pepper. Reserve 21/2 teaspoons of this mixture.

3. To the remaining spice mixture, add 1 tablespoon oil and 2 tablespoons lemon juice. Cut the tofu into cubes of about 3/4-inches and pat dry. Add to the spice mixture and add the chickpeas. Stir and let it rest for 10 minutes.

4. In a single layer, spread the tofu and chickpeas on a greased baking sheet. Roast for 20 minutes, on the lower rack, stirring halfway through cooking.

5. Meanwhile, add the reserved spice mixture to the large bowl. Add the remain- ing oil and lemon juice. Add the kale, and rub with hands to reduce in half. Add the cucumber and bell pepper, tossing to mix well.

6. Serve the salad on a bowl and top with the roasted tofu and chickpeas.

Nutrition Facts:

Per Serving; Calories 355; Fat 20.3g; Carbohydrates 32.6g; Protein 16g; Fiber 8.5g; Sodium: 631mg;

20.   Spaghetti with Garlic Shrimp & Buttered Kale

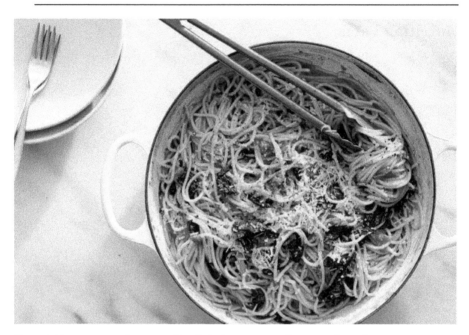

Prep Time: 15 minutes Cook Time: 15 minutes Servings: 4

Ingredients

8 oz. whole-grain spaghetti

10 oz. shrimp, peeled & then deveined

1/2 teaspoon freshly ground black pepper

1/4 teaspoon salt

1 tablespoon extra-virgin olive oil

4 large cloves garlic, sliced

1/4 teaspoon red pepper

1 teaspoon dried parsley

2 teaspoon lemon zest

2 tablespoons unsalted butter

4 cups stemmed kale, sliced finely

1 red finger chile pepper, sliced thinly

Directions

1. Cook the spaghetti according to instructions on the package; but cook it al

dente and then drain.

2. While it cooks, season the shrimp with salt and pepper and toss to coat. Heat up the olive oil and sauté the garlic and then add the parsley, and the pepper flakes. Cook and stir for several seconds until fragrant.

3. Add the shrimp and sauté for 4 minutes, stirring frequently until pinkish. Re- move to a plate and cover.

4. Add butter to same skillet and then add the kale. Cook for a minute until wilt- ed. Add the pasta, the shrimp mixture and the chile pepper. Stir thoroughly to mix.

Nutrition Facts:

Per Serving; Calories 384; Fat 12g; Carbohydrates 51g; Protein 2 3g; Fiber 7g; Sodium 209mg; Cholesterol 115mg

21.   Chilli Con Carne

Prep Time: 30minutes Cook Time: 1 hr. 30 minutes Servings: 4

Ingredients

1 red onion

3 garlic cloves

2 bird's eye chillies

1 tablespoon of extra virgin olive oil

1 tablespoon of ground turmeric

1 tablespoon of ground cumin

14 ounce lean minced beef

¾ cup of red wine 1 red pepper

2-14oz tins chopped tomatoes 1 tablespoon of tomato purée

5 oz. can kidney beans 1 tablespoon of cocoa powder

11/4 cup of beef stock

2 tablespoons of parsley

2 tablespoons of coriander

51/2 oz. buckwheat

Directions

1. Chop the red onion, clove garlic and chilies finely, take out the core of the red pepper, remove the seeds and cut into pieces, chop the coriander and the parsley.

2. Add oil to pan and fry the onion, garlic and chilli for a couple of minutes over medium heat. Add the spices and cook an

additional minute. Add the minced beef, increase the heat and cook until brown. Add the red wine and cook until it reduces by half.

3. Now add the red pepper, the tomatoes, the puree, kidney beans, cocoa and the stock; lower heat and let it simmer for an hour. Add a little water, if necessary.

4. Once cooked, add the chopped herbs, turn off heat and stir.

5. Cook the buckwheat and serve with the chilli.

Nutrition Facts:

Per Serving; Calories 417; Fat 15g; Carbohydrates 42g; Protein 3 3g; Fiber 8g; Sodium 265mg; Cholesterol 0mg

22.   Lamb, Butternut Squash and Date Tagine

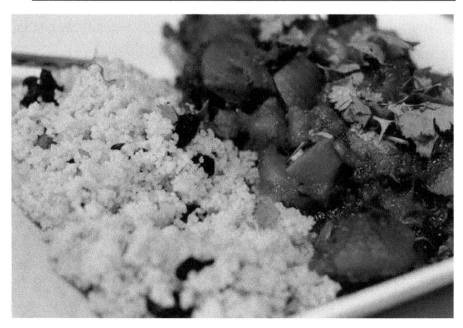

Preparation time: 5 minutes Cooking time: 1 hour and 15 minutes Servings: 4

Ingredients:

2 Tsps. coconut oil

1 Red onion, chopped

2cm ginger, grated

3 Garlic cloves, crushed or grated

1 teaspoon chili flakes (or to taste)

2 tsp. cumin seeds

2 teaspoons ground turmeric 1 cinnamon stick

800g lamb neck fillet, cut into

2cm chunks

1/2 tsp. salt 100g Medjool dates, pitted and sliced

400g Tin chopped berries, and half of a can of plain water 500g
Butternut squash, chopped into 1cm cubes

400g Tin chickpeas, drained

2 tsp. fresh coriander (and extra for garnish) Buckwheat,
Couscous, flatbread or rice to function

Directions: Pre heat the oven to 140C. Drizzle roughly 2 tbsps.
coconut oil into a large ovenproof saucepan or cast- iron casserole
dish. Add the chopped onion and cook on a gentle heat, with the
lid for around five minutes, until the onions are softened but not
too brown. Insert the grated ginger and garlic, chili, cumin,
cinnamon, and garlic. Stir well and cook 1 minute with off the lid.
Add a dash of water when it becomes too humid. Add from the
lamb balls. Stir to coat the beef from the spices and onions,
and then add the salt chopped meats and berries and roughly half
of a can of plain water (100-200ml). Bring the tagine into the boil
and put the lid and put on your skillet for about 1 hour and fifteen
minutes. Add the chopped butternut squash and drained
chickpeas. Stir everything to- gether, place the lid back and go
back to the oven to the last half an hour of cook- ing. When the
tagine is able to remove from the oven and then stir fry
throughout the chopped coriander.

Nutrition Facts:

Calories: 317 Total Fat: 18 g Total Carbohydrates: 14 g Protein: 22 g

23.   Prawn Arrabbiata

Preparation time: 15 minutes Cooking time: 35 minutes

Ingredients:

125-150 g Beef or cooked prawns (Ideally king prawns)

65 g Buckwheat pasta

1 tablespoon extra-virgin coconut oil

Arrabbiata sauce

40 g Red onion, finely chopped

1 Garlic clove, finely chopped

30 g celery, thinly sliced

1 Bird's eye chili, finely chopped

1 tsp. Dried mixed veggies 1 tsp. extra virgin coconut oil

2 Tablespoon White wine (optional)

400 Gram tinned chopped berries

1 tbsp. Chopped parsley

Directions: Fry the garlic, onion, celery, and peppermint and peppermint blossoms at the oil over moderate-low heat for 1- 2 weeks. Turn up the heat to medium, bring the wine and cook 1 second. Add the berries and leave the sauce simmer over moderate-low heat for 20 to half an hour, until it's a great rich texture. In the event you're feeling that the sauce is becoming too thick, simply put in just a very little water. As the sauce is cooking, attract a bowl of water to the boil and then cook the pasta as per the package directions. Once cooked to your dish, drain, then toss with the olive oil and also maintain at the pan before needed. If you're utilizing raw prawns, put them into your sauce and cook for a further 3 - 4 minutes, till they've turned opaque and pink, and then add the parsley and function. If you're using cooked prawns, insert them using the skillet, and then bring the sauce to the boil and then function. Add the cooked pasta into the sauce, then mix thoroughly but lightly and function.

Nutrition Facts:

Calories: 415 Total Fat: 10 g Total Carbohydrates: 57 g Protein: 23 g

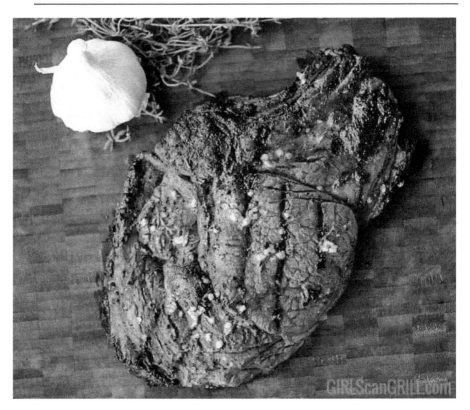

Preparation time: 30 minutes:

Ingredients:

5g parsley, finely chopped

100g potatoes, peeled and cut into 2cm dice

50g Lettuce, chopped

1 tbsp. extra virgin coconut oil

50g Red onion, chopped into circles

1 garlic clove, finely chopped 1

20 - 150g

3.5cm thick beef noodle beef or 2cm-thick sirloin beef

40ml Red wine

150ml Beef inventory

1 tsp. tomato purée

1 tsp. corn flour, dissolved in 1 tablespoon water

Direction: Heating the oven to 220°C Put the sausage in a saucepan of boiling water, then return to the boil and then cook 4 minutes, then empty. Put in a skillet with 1 tbsp. of the oil and then roast in the oven for 4 − 5 minutes. Twist the berries every 10 minutes to ensure even cooking. After cooking, re- move from the oven, sprinkle with the chopped parsley, and mix well. Fry the onion 1 tsp. of the oil over a moderate heat for 5 minutes until tender and well caramelized. Maintain heat. Steam the kale for 2 - 3 minutes. Stir the garlic lightly in 1/2 tsp. of oil for 1 minute until tender but not colored. Insert the spinach and simmer for a further 1—two minutes, until tender. Maintain heat. Heat ovenproof skillet until smoking then laid the beef from 1/2 a tsp. of the oil. Then fry from the skillet over a moderate-high temperature in accordance with just how you would like your beef done. If you prefer your beef moderate, it'd be wise to sear the beef and also transfer the pan into a toaster place in 220°C/petrol 7 and then finish the cooking which manner to your prescribed occasions. Remove the meat from the pan and put aside to break. Add your wine into the skillet to bring any meat up residue. Bubble to decrease the wine by half an hour until syrupy, along with a flavor that is concentrated. Insert the inventory and tomato purée into the beef pan and bring to the boil, add the corn flour paste to thicken your sauce, then adding it only a little at a time till you've got your preferred consistency. Stir in just about anyone of those juices out of the dinner that is rested and serve with the roasted lettuce, celery, onion rings, and red berry sauce.

Nutrition Facts:

Calories: 416 Total Fat: 13 g Total Carbohydrates: 39 g Protein: 35 g

25.   Fruity Curry Chicken Salad

Preparation time: 10 minutes Cooking time: 10 minutes Servings: 8

Ingredients

4 skinless, boneless chicken pliers - cooked and diced

1 tsp. celery, diced

4 green onions, sliced

1 golden delicious apple peeled, cored and diced

1/3 cup golden raisins

1/3 cup seedless green grapes, halved

1/2 cup sliced toasted pecans

1/8 tsp. Ground black pepper

1/2 tsp. curry powder

3/4 cup light mayonnaise

Directions:

In a big bowl combine the chicken, onion, celery, apple, celery, celery, pecans, pepper, curry powder, and carrot. Mix altogether.

Nutrition Facts:

Calories: 156 Total Fat: 6 g Total Carbohydrates: 10 g Protein: 14 g

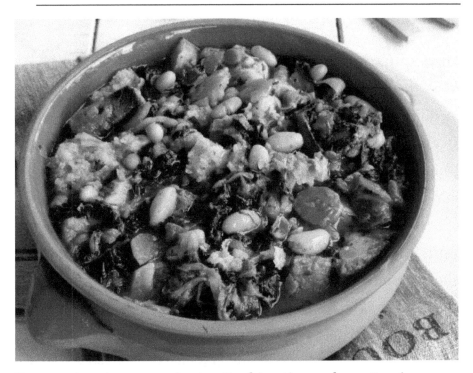

Preparation time: 20 minutes Cooking time: 1 hour Servings: 2

Ingredients:

1 lb ground Italian sausage

1 1/4 tsp. crushed red pepper flakes

4 pieces bacon, cut into

½ inch bits

1 big onion, diced

1 tbsp. minced garlic

5 (13.75 oz) can chicken broth

6 celery, thinly chopped

1 cup thick cream

1/4 bunch fresh spinach, tough stems removed

Directions:

Cook that the Italian sausage and red pepper flakes in a pot on medium-high heat until crumbly, browned, with no longer pink, 10 to 15minutes. Drain and put aside. Cook the bacon at the exact Dutch oven over moderate heat until crispy, about 10 minutes. Drain leaving a couple of tablespoons of drippings together with all the bacon at the bottom of the toaster. Stir in the garlic and onions cook until onions are ten- der and translucent, about 5 minutes. Pour the chicken broth to the pot with the onion and bacon mix; contribute to a boil on high temperature. Add the berries, and boil until fork-tender, about 20 minutes. Reduce heat to moderate and stir in the cream and also the cooked sausage – heat throughout. Mix the lettuce to the soup before serving.

Nutrition Facts:

Calories: 403 Total Fat: 24 g Cholesterol: 66 mg Total Carbohydrates: 32 g

27.   Farinata with Zucchini and Shallot

Preparation time: 15 minutes Cooking time: 40 minutes Servings: 4

Ingredients: 400 ml of water

125 g of chickpea flour

60 g of Evo oil

8 g of salt

1 zucchini

1 shallot

Directions: Put the water in a container; gradually add the flour mixing with the whisk to avoid creating lumps. Add the oil, salt, chopped shallot, zucchini cut into rounds and keep stirring until the mixture is well blended. Pour it all into a round baking tray greased with a drizzle of oil. Cook at 250° for 30-40 minutes. Once it's out of the oven, let it cool before you serve it.

Nutrition Facts:

Calories: 129 Total Fat: 6 g Sodium: 250 mg Potassium: 195 mg Total Carbohydrates: 13 g Protein: 5 g

28.   Stuffed with Vegetables

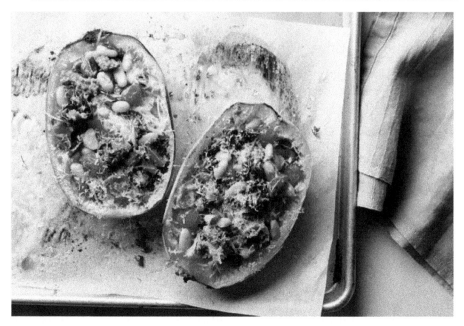

Preparation time: 5 minutes Cooking time: 15 minutes Servings: 2

Ingredients:

4 large spoons of chickpea flour

2 level teaspoons of powdered vegetable broth preparation

Sunflower seed oil

300 g mixed vegetables already cooked (e.g. a ratatouille or any other vegetable mix)

Directions:

Mix with a whisk the chickpea flour and the powdered cube, adding water to obtain a rather liquid but still creamy consistency. Swirl the vegetables with a little sunflower oil and, once heated, pour the batter. For a crispier omelet, the batter layer must be only a few mm thick (maximum one cm, when the filling is abundant). Cook over low heat on one side until the top has thickened as well. At this point turn with the method you prefer and complete the cooking on the other side.

Nutrition Facts:

Calories: 171 Total Fat: 5 g Sodium: 225 mg Potassium: 390 mg Total Carbohydrates: 25 g Protein: 5 g

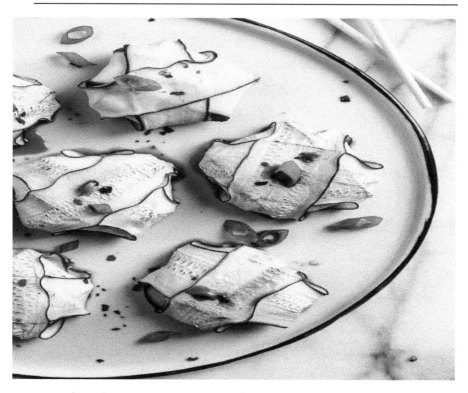

Preparation time: 15 minutes Cooking time: 1 hour Servings: 4

Ingredients:

2 zucchini

1 vegan puff pastry for savory pies

8 pitted green olives Sunflower seeds

1 onion Pepper Oil

Directions: Cut the zucchini into thin slices, put them in the non-stick pan with a drizzle of oil (very little) and simmer them with the lid for about 30 minutes, until well cooked. Roll out the puff pastry and divide it into 4 parts. Chop the olives; add the chopped onion and some sunflower seeds. In a small cup place some zucchini (just enough for a dumpling) and add a quarter of the chopped olives, mix and place on the puff pastry. Add pepper and a drizzle of oil. Repeat the operation for the 4 dumplings, then close them by joining the corners and bake for 30 minutes. You can also use other vegetables instead of zucchini.

Nutrition Fatcs:

Calories: 240 Total Fat: 8 g Total Carbohydrates: 26 g Protein: 10

30. Sponge Beans with Onion

Preparation time: 5 minutes Cooking time: 1 hour and 30 minutes Servings: 2

Ingredients:

250 g boiled Spanish beans

1 red onion

1 tablespoon parsley Salt

2 tablespoons of oil

1 teaspoon of apple vinegar

1 teaspoon of dried oregano or

5 fresh oregano leaves

Directions:

Cut the onion into thin slices and cook it for a minute with a tablespoon of water in the microwave at full power. Combine all the ingredients in a bowl and leave to rest a couple of hours before serving, stirring a couple of times so that the beans take on the flavour of the sea- soning.

Nutrition Facts:

Calories: 250 Total Fat: 7 g Total Carbohydrates: 36 g Protein: 5 g

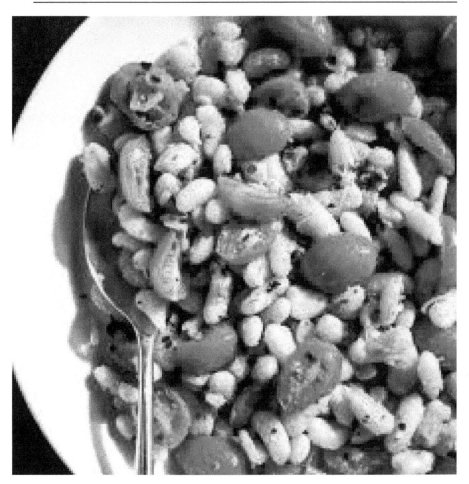

Preparation time: 5 minutes Cooking time: 25 minutes Servings: 1

Ingredients:

2 cloves of garlic, minced

2 sage leaves

2 tablespoons of extra virgin olive oil

Boiled cannellini beans Fresh well ripe tomatoes

Salt and pepper

Directions: Cook for 2-3 minutes in a pan with oil, garlic and sage.

Then add the tomatoes, cut into segments, and let them brown for a couple of minutes. Add the beans, salt and pepper to taste, stir. Cook in a covered pot for 20 minutes, checking and turning occasionally. Serve hot.

Nutrition Fatcs:

Calories: 320 Total Fat: 7 g Total Carbohydrates: 54 g Protein: 18 g

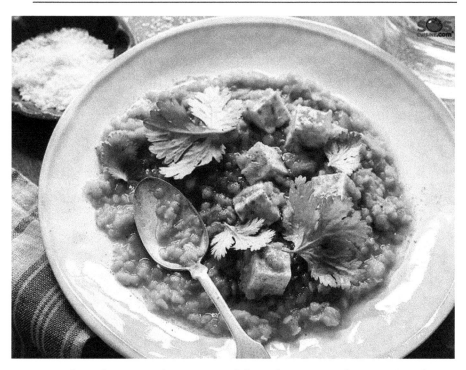

Preparation time: 5 minutes Cooking time: 30 minutes Servings: 2

Ingredients:

200 g of tofu cake

Soy sauce (shoyu)

Extra virgin olive oil

Onion Sprig of rosemary

2 tablespoons of chopped chili pepper

50 g of red lentils Vegetable stock Breadcrumbs

Directions:

Marinate the diced tofu for half an hour in the soy sauce, adding a little water to cover it. In the meantime, boil the red lentils, washed in the vegetable stock for about 20 minutes, until they are soft enough and the stock has dried a bit. Sauté 2 tablespoons of chili pepper then diced onion and rosemary in olive oil until the onion is golden brown. Add the tofu with some of the marinating shoyu and after a few minutes also the lentils with very little broth. Let everything shrink with the lid and over low heat and to thicken add 2 table- spoons of breadcrumbs.

Nutrition Facts:

Calories: 63 Total Fat: 3 g Total Carbohydrates: 2 g Fiber: 1 g Protein: 8 g

33. Cauliflower Fried Rice With Crispy Tofu

Prep Time: 15 minutes Cook Time: 15 minutes

Ingredients

Baked Tofu: 15 oz. extra firm tofu, pressed & cubed

1 tablespoon of Extra Virgin olive oil

1 tablespoon cornstarch

1 tablespoon soy sauce Cauliflower Fried Rice:

1 medium cauliflower head, cut into florets Olive oil

2 garlic cloves, minced

1 ginger knob, grated

2cups of frozen peas and carrots

Soy sauce Sriracha

Sesame oil

3 beaten eggs

Green onions

Instructions

1. Preheat oven to 450F.

2. Combine the olive oil, tofu, cornstarch and soy sauce in a bowl, mix well and place on a paper-lined baking sheet. Bake 30 minutes, flipping half way through cooking.

3. Place florets in a food processor until they are rice-like in consistency.

4. Add olive oil to pan and heat and then add the ginger, garlic, peas and car- rots. Stir and cook and then add the cauliflower, and the Sriracha. Cook to just soften the cauliflower for 2 minutes.

5. Make a well in the centre of the pan and then add the sesame oil and the eggs, pulling eggs gently to make scrambled eggs. Stir the cooked scrambled eggs with the rest of the ingredients.

6. Serve, topped with green onions and more Sriracha.

Nutrition Facts:

Calories per serving: 297 Serves: 4

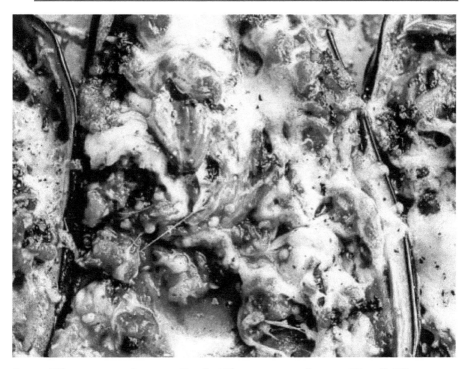

Prep Time: 15 minutes Cook Time: 40 minutes Total Time: 55 minutes

Ingredients:

2 large eggplants, halved lengthwise 2 tablespoons of extra virgin olive oil 1 yellow onion, finely chopped 1 pound Italian sausage casing removed, 1/4 cup of fresh parsley, finely chopped 1/2 teaspoon of dried oregano 1/2 teaspoon of dried thyme 4 cloves of garlic, minced Salt and pepper to taste 1 cup of warm water 1 cup of mozzarella cheese, shredded **Instructions** 1. First, preheat oven to 400°F.

2. Scoop out the pulp from the halved eggplants, chop into pieces and set aside. Transfer eggplant shells into a baking sheet halved side up, season with salt and pepper and set aside. 3. Next, heat up olive oil in a large sized skillet over medium heat, add onions and eggplant pulp to the skillet and cook for 2-3 minutes, stirring frequently. 4. Mash Italian sausage with clean hands and add to the skillet, stir and then add the parsley, oregano, thyme, garlic, salt and pepper and cook for 5 minutes until done. 5. Taste the mixture and adjust seasoning as preferred. Remove from heat and set aside to cool. 6. Next, gently stuff the eggplant shells with the sausage mixture. Pour the warm water around the baking sheet then transfer to the oven to bake. 7. Cook for 20-25 minutes until the eggplant is tender. Afterwards, remove from the oven and drizzle cheese over each eggplant. 8. Place baking sheet back into the oven and cook for 5 minutes until cheese is melted. 9. Remove from oven and cool for a few minutes before serving, enjoy!

Nutrition Facts:

Calories per Serving: 603 Serves: 4 (1 stuffed eggplant each)

35.   Tuscan Carrot Bean Stew

Prep time: 10 minutes Cook time: 40 minutes Servings: 1

INGREDIENTS

40 grams of buckwheat

1 tbsp of roughly chopped parsley

50 grams of kale, roughly chopped 200 grams of tinned mixed beans

1 tsp of tomato purée

400 grams of tin chopped Italian tomatoes 200 ml of vegetable stock

1 tsp of herbes de Provence (Optional) half bird's eye chilli, finely chopped 1 finely chopped garlic clove

30 grams of celery, trimmed and finely chopped

30 grams of peeled and chopped carrot

50 grams of finely chopped red onion

1 tbsp of extra virgin olive oil

INSTRUCTIONS

1. Gently fry the onion, celery, carrot, chilli (if using), garlic and herbs in hot oil over a low–medium heat in a medium saucepan until the onion is soft.

2. Add the tomato purée, vegetable stock and tomatoes and bring to a boil. Pour in beans and simmer about 30 minutes.

3. Add chopped kale and cook for additional 6 to 10 minutes, until kale is soft, add in chopped parsley.

4. Cook the buckwheat the way instructed in packet directions, drain. Serve cooked buckwheat noodles with bean stew.

Nutrition Facts:

kcal: 306 Net carbs: 29 g Fat: 12.23g Fiber: 15 g Protein:9.91g

36. Baked Cod Marinated In Miso With Greens

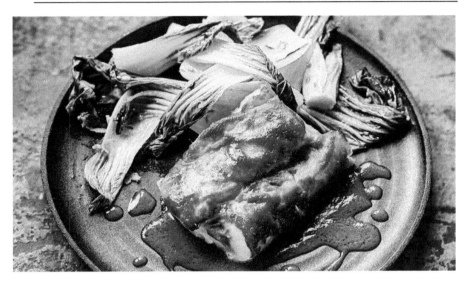

Prep time: 50 minutes Cook time: 25 minutes Servings: 1

INGREDIENTS

1 tsp of ground turmeric

1⁄4 cup of buckwheat (40g)

1 tbsp of soy sauce

2 tbsp of roughly chopped parsley, (5g)

1 tsp of sesame seeds

3⁄4 cup of roughly chopped kale, (50g)

3⁄8 cup of green beans (60g)

1 tsp of finely chopped fresh ginger

1 finely chopped Thai chili

2 finely chopped garlic cloves

3/8 cup of sliced celery, (40g)

1/8 cup of sliced red onion, (20g)

1 x 7-oz of skinless cod fillet (200g)

1 tbsp of extra virgin olive oil

1 tbsp of mirin

(20g)

3 1/2 tsp of miso

Instructions

1. Mix together 1 tsp of olive oil, miso and mirin. Rub the cod all over with the mix- ture and let it marinate for half hour.

2. Preheat the oven to 425 degrees F. Once you are done marinating, place the cod in the oven and bake for 10 minutes.

3. While the cod is cooking, pour the remaining olive oil in a large frying pan and heat over medium heat. Stir-fry the onion in the hot oil for a few minutes, add the ginger, celery, kale, garlic, green beans, and chili. Cook stirring frequently and toss- ing until the kale is cooked through and tender. Add a few drops of water to pan if needed.

4. Cook the buckwheat along with turmeric the way instructed in package instruction.

5. Add the soy sauce, parsley and sesame seeds to the stir-fry. Serve fish with the stir-fry and buckwheat.

Nutrition Facts:

kcal: 500 Net carbs: 65 g Fat: 17.26g Fiber: 22 g

37. Mushrooms With Buckwheat Kasha And Olives

Prep time: 5 minutes Cook time: 20 minutes Servings: 4

INGREDIENTS

1/4 cup of chopped parsley

1/2 cup of black olives sliced

8 ounces of baby bella mushrooms 1 tbsp of olive oil 1 tbsp of almond butter

1 cup of buckwheat groats toasted 2 teaspoon salt 2 tbsp of soy sauce

INSTRUCTIONS

1. Add 2 cups of water, buckwheat, butter and salt in a pot. Bring mixture to a boil, turn heat down and simmer for 20 minutes with the lid on.

2. Add the olive oil to pan over medium high heat. Add in the mushrooms and fry about 10-15 minutes or until lightly browned.

3. Combine together the mushrooms/buckwheat mix, olives, soy sauce and parsley Mix In a large bowl.

Nutrition Facts:

kcal: 235 Net carbs: 34 g Fat: 10.26g Fiber: 8g Protein:7.7g

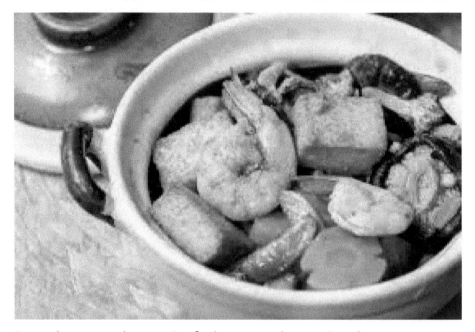

Prep time: 10 minutes Cook time: 15 minutes Servings: 5

INGREDIENTS

1 tbsp of good-quality miso paste

20 grams of sushi ginger, chopped

50 grams of cooked water chestnuts, drained

50 grams of rice noodles

100 grams of chopped firm tofu

100 grams of raw tiger prawns

50 grams of bean sprouts

50 grams of broccoli, cut into small florets

1/2 carrot, cut into matchsticks

500 ml of fresh chicken stock, or made with

1 cube Juice of 1/2 lime Small handful of coriander, stalks finely chopped (10g)

Small handful of parsley, stalks finely chopped (10g)

1 crushed star anise, or 1/4 tsp of ground anise

1 tsp of tomato purée

INSTRUCTIONS

1. In a large pan, add the chicken stock, star anise, tomato purée, parsley stalks, lime juice and coriander stalks and bring mixture to a simmer, about 10 minutes. 2. Cook the rice noodles according to packet instructions, drain. 3. Add cooked noodles, broccoli, tofu, carrot, prawns, and water chestnuts and gently simmer until the vegetables and prawns are cooked. Turn heat off and stir in the miso paste and sushi ginger. Serve with a sprinkle of coriander and parsley.

Nutrition Facts:

kcal: 139 Net carbs: 13 g Fat: 3.9g Fiber: 2.8 g Protein: 11g

39. Buckwheat Kasha With Onions Mushrooms

Prep time: 10 minutes Cook time: 30 minutes Servings: 4

INGREDIENTS

A small bunch of dill, chopped Salt and freshly ground black pepper

250 grams of brown mushrooms

1 tbsp of olive oil A small bunch of parsley, less than dill, chopped

2 tbsp of butter, divided

3 small red onions, thinly sliced

450 ml of chicken stock or vegetable broth (a bit less than 2 cups)

1 egg

150 grams of roasted buckwheat groats

INSTRUCTIONS

1. Lightly whisk the egg in a bowl. Mix in the buckwheat until well mixed.

2. Heat a non stick pan over medium heat, add buckwheat and cook until all the corns are separated and dry, about 3-4 minutes.

3. Transfer the buckwheat to a small saucepan. Add in the stock or broth and bring to a boil, reduce heat and let it simmer for 15 minutes or there about until stock has been absorbed and the buckwheat is soft.

4. Heat the olive oil with 1 tbsp. butter in the pan on low heat; add onions and cook, stirring often for 15 minutes or until tender and golden brown. You can add a few splash of water in between so the onion won't catch.

5. Add in the mushrooms and cook for additional 5-7 minutes or until withered and cooked; season with salt and pepper.

6. Add in buckwheat and stir to coat well. Stir in the remaining butter. Add in chopped parsley and dill. Serve with some green salad.

Nutrition Facts:

kcal: 223 Net carbs: 19 g Fat: 12g Fiber: 3 g Protein: 8g

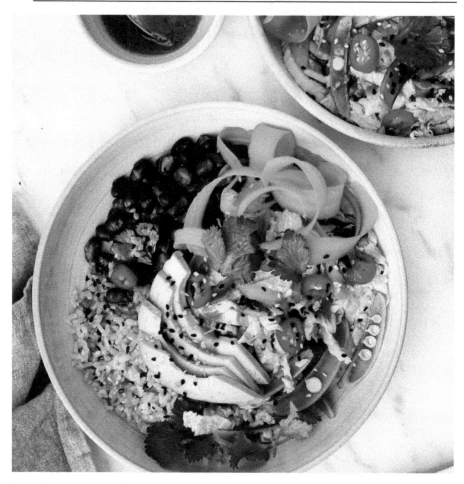

Ready time: 5 minutes Serving: 4

INGREDIENTS:

Sea salt (Himalayan, Celtic Grey, or Redmond Real Salt)

1 lime juice

1 avocado

8 butter lettuce leaves or romaine, these make lovely cups Small handful of chopped cilantro

¼ cup of red onion, minced

1 15-oz can of Adzuki beans, drained and rinsed Red pepper flakes (optional)

INSTRUCTIONS 1. In a bowl, mash together the red onion and beans. Add chopped cilantro, stir to combine. 2. Spoon the mash beans into lettuce cups and add diced avocado to the top with lime juice; season with red pepper flakes and salt.

Nutrition Facts:

kcal: 118 Net carbs: 6 g Fat: 8g Fiber: 6 g Protein: 2.69g

41.   Baked Salmon

Prep time: 15-20 minutes Cook time: 10 minutes Servings: 1

INGREDIENTS

1/4 Juice of a lemon

1 tsp of ground turmeric

1 tsp of extra virgin olive oil

125-150 grams of skinned salmon

For the spicy celery

1 tbsp of chopped parsley

100 ml vegetable or chicken stock

130 grams of tomato, cut into 8 wedges

1 tsp of mild curry powder

150 grams of celery, cut into 2 cm lengths

1 finely chopped Bird's eye chilli

1 cm finely chopped fresh ginger

1 Garlic clove, finely chopped

60 grams of tinned green lentils

40 grams of red onion, finely chopped

1 tsp of extra virgin olive oil

Instructions

1. Preheat your oven to 200C / gas mark 6.

For the spicy celery

2. Heat the olive oil over medium–low heat in a hot frying pan; add the garlic,

onion, chilli, ginger and celery. Gently sauté for about 2–3 minutes, then pour in

the curry powder and sauté for another minute.

3. Add the tomatoes, lentils and vegetable or chicken stock and gently simmer for

7-10 minutes.

4. Meanwhile, mix the lemon juice, oil and turmeric and rub all over the salmon.

5. Place seasoned salmon onto a baking tray and cook in the preheated oven for

8–10 minutes. Stir the parsley into the celery mixture and serve over the salmon.

Nutrition Information:

kcal: 340

Net carbs: 25g

Fat: 11.9g

Fiber: 7.5g

Protein: 41 g

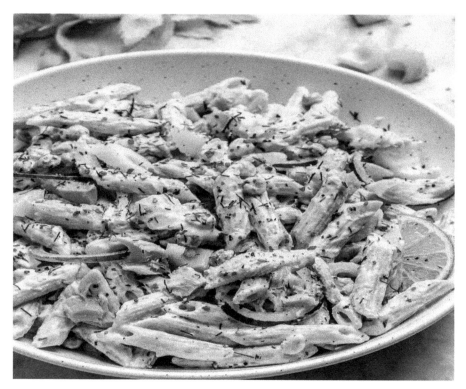

Servings: 1

Ingredients

20 grams of pine nuts

1 tbsp of extra virgin olive oil

10 olives

1/2 diced avocado

8 cherry tomatoes, halved

Small handful of basil leaves

A large handful of rocket

50 grams of buckwheat pasta (cooked according to the packet instructions)

Instructions

1. Cook the buckwheat noodles according to the packet instructions.

2. Combine together the cooked pasta, olive oil, olives, diced avocado, basil leaves,

tomatoes and rocket in a bowl. Serve noodles on a plate and spread the pine nuts

over top.

Nutrition Information:

kcal: 290; Net carbs: 7.2; Fat: 31.52g; Protein: 3.92 g

43.   Beef Red Onion Potatoes Burgers

Prep time: 15 minutes Ready time: 30 minutes Servings: 1

Ingredients

(Optional) 1 gherkin

10 grams of rocket

30 grams of tomato, sliced

150 grams of red onion, sliced into rings

10 grams of sliced or grated Cheddar cheese

1 unpeeled garlic clove

1 tsp of dried rosemary

1 tsp of olive oil

150 grams of sweet potatoes, peel and cut into 1cm thick chips

1 tsp of olive oil

1 tsp of finely chopped parsley

15 grams of finely chopped red onion

125 grams of lean minced beef (5% fat)

Instructions

1. Preheat the oven to 450 f.

2. Toss sweet potato chips with the oil, garlic clove and rosemary. Add to the bak-

ing pan and roast in the oven until nice and crispy, about 30 minutes.

3. Mix the minced beef with parsley and onion. Mold using your hands into an even

patty or use a pastry cutters and mold, if you have one.

4. Heat the olive oil over medium heat in a hot frying pan; add onion rings towards

one side of the frying pan and the burger over the other. Cook onion rings to your

liking and burger for about 6 minutes per side until burger is cooked through.

5. Top the burger with the red onion and cheese, transfer to the preheated oven

until cheese is melted. Remove from the oven and top with the tomato, gherkin

and rocket. Serve along the fries.

Nutrition Information:

kcal: 406

Net carbs: 35g

Fat: 17g

Fiber: 5.5 g

Protein: 32.17 g

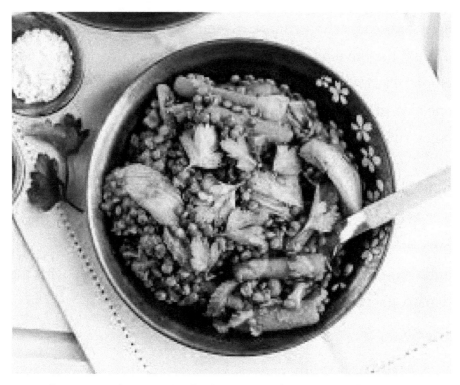

Prep time: 40 minutes Cook time: 60 minutes Servings: 1

Ingredients

20 grams of rocket

1 tbsp of parsley, chopped

50 grams of kale, roughly chopped

220 ml of vegetable stock

75 grams of puy lentils

1 tsp of thyme (dry or fresh)

1 tsp of paprika

40 grams of carrots, peeled and thinly sliced

40 grams of thinly sliced Celery

1 finely chopped garlic clove

40 grams of thinly sliced red onion

2 tsp of extra virgin olive oil

8 cherry tomatoes, halved

Instructions

1. Heat the oven to 120 C

2. Roast the tomatoes in the oven in a small baking pan for 35–45 minutes.

3. Heat 1 teaspoon of the olive oil over low–medium heat in a saucepan. Add the onion, celery, garlic, and carrot slices and cook for 1 to 2 minutes until tender. Add the thyme and paprika and cook for extra 1 minute.

4. Add lentils and Vegetable stock into the pan, and bring to the boil. Turn heat down and simmer with the lid on for 20 minutes. Add a splash of water if needed and make sure you stir 5-7 minutes intervals.

5. Add in kale and keep cooking for another 10 minutes. Stir in the roasted tomatoes and parsley. Serve along the rocket and drizzle top with the remaining olive oil.

Nutrition Information:

kcal: 283 Net carbs: 45g Fat: 17g Fiber: 9.6g Protein: 5.71 g

45.Buckwheat Noodles With Stir-Fry Prawn

Prep time: 10 minutes Cook time: 10 minutes Servings: 1

Ingredients

5g lovage or celery leaves

100 ml of chicken stock

50 g roughly chopped kale

75g chopped green beans

40g trimmed and sliced celery

20g sliced red onions

1 tsp of finely chopped fresh ginger

1 finely chopped bird's eye chilli

1 finely chopped garlic clove

75g of soba buckwheat noodles

2 tsp of extra virgin olive oil

2 tsp soy sauce or soy sauce

150g of shelled raw king prawns, deveined

Instructions

1. Heat 1 tsp of the oil and 1 tsp. of the soy sauce over high heat in a frying pan, add

prawns and cook about 2–3 minutes. Set prawns aside in a plate. Prepare the pan

for another use.

2. Cook the buckwheat noodles the way instructed in package instruction. Drain and set aside.

3. Meanwhile, heat the remaining oil over medium–high and fry the red onion, garlic, ginger, chilli, celery and kale and beans for 2–3 minutes. Add in the chicken stock and bring to a boil, simmer for 1 to 2 minute until the vegetables are soft but still firm to the bite.

4. Add buckwheat noodles, prawns, noodles and lovage to the pan, bring to a boil. Turn heat off and serve.

46.Baked Mackerel Fillets With Potatoes

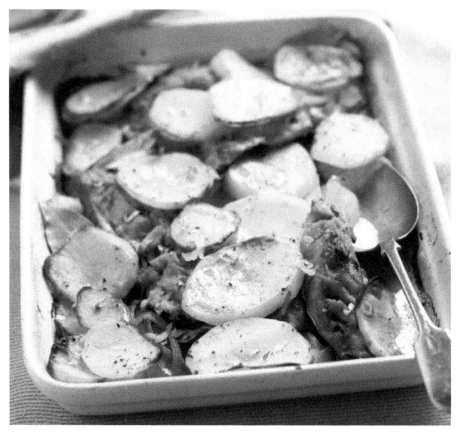

Prep time: 5 minutes Cook time: 25 minutes Servings: 4

Ingredients

1/4 pint of vegetable stock

1 tbsp of olive oil

7-ounces of cherry tomatoes

2-ounces of pitted black olives

11-ounces of mackerel fillets

1 lemon

2 sweet potatoes, chopped

2 leeks, chopped

Instructions

1. Heat-up the oven to 375 F. Place the leeks and sweet potatoes in a roasting pan.

Add the stock and drizzle with 1 tablespoon of olive oil.

2. Place pan in the oven and roast for 15-20 minutes until potatoes are soft. Add the

cherry tomatoes, mackerel fillets and black olives. Top with a squeeze of lemon

juice and roast for extra 10 minutes.

Nutrition Information:

kcal: 230; Net carbs: 21g; Fat: 7.4g; Fiber: 4g; Protein: 18.22 g

47.Baked Broccoli Macaroni And Cheese

Prep Time: 10minutes Cook Time: 30minutes Servings: 8

Ingredients

12 oz. pasta

1 1/2 tablespoons of melted butter

1/4 cup of onion, minced

1/4 cup flour

2 cups skim milk

1 cup broth

2 cups of low fat sharp cheddar cheese

Salt and freshly ground pepper to taste

12 oz. fresh broccoli florets

1/4 cup of seasoned bread crumbs

Directions

1. Add the pasta and broccoli in a pot, add some salt and water and cook for about 2 minutes until slightly cooked.

2. Preheat oven to 375°F.

3. Melt butter in a skillet; add the onion and sauté 2 minutes on low heat. Add the flour and cook 1 minute. Add the milk. Broth and stir. Raise heat and bring to a boil. Cook sauce until thickened and then add salt and pepper to season.

4. Remove thickened sauce from heat, add the cheese, mix to melt and add salt and pepper as needed. Add the slightly cooked pasta and broccoli and mix thoroughly.

5. Transfer to a greased baking dish; add grated cheese on top. Add the breadcrumbs. Spritz with oil.

6. Bake 20 minutes, then broil for about 2 minutes to ensure a golden breadcrumbs.

Nutrition Facts:

Per Serving; Calories 315; Fat 10g; Carbohydrates 44g; Protein 18g; Fiber 6g; Sodium: 216mg; Cholesterol: 7mg

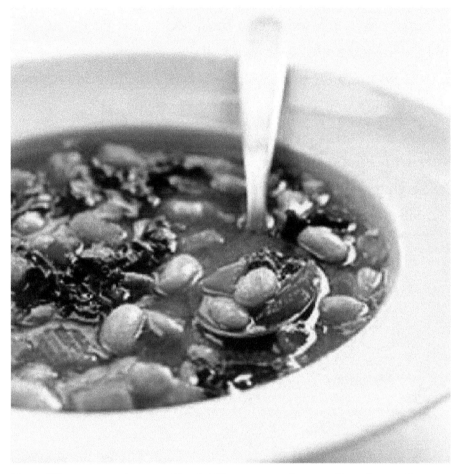

Prep Time: 20 minutes Cook Time: 40 minutes Servings: 6

Ingredients

1 tablespoon olive oil

1 cup diced red onion

1/4 cup diced celery

1/2 cup diced carrot

1 teaspoon dried thyme

4 medium cloves garlic, minced

1/4 teaspoon crushed red pepper flakes

1/2 teaspoon kosher salt

1/4 teaspoon ground black pepper

1 (15-oz) can kidney beans, drained (about 1 1/2 cups)

1 (15-oz.) can cannellini or beans, drained (about 1 1/2 cups)

1 (15-ounce) can lima beans, drained (about 1 1/2 cups)

2 cups reduced sodium vegetable broth

1 bay leaf

2 5-inch sprigs rosemary

1 small bunch kale, cut in pieces (about 4 cups)

Salt and pepper to taste

Directions:

1. Heat the olive oil in oil and once hot, add the onions, celery and carrots.

Cook and stir for 5 minutes and when it's tender, add the thyme, black pepper and salt, stir and then add the beans. Pour in the broth, add the rosemary and the bay leaf. Stir all together. Raise the heat to medium high and bring mixture to a boil.

2. Now lower heat and let it simmer for 25 minutes or thereabouts, to thicken the stew. Add the kale and cook for 3 minutes to wilt.

3. Take out the sprigs of rosemary and the bay leaf. Adjust seasonings as needed.

4. Enjoy as is or serve over quinoa or brown rice, drizzled with olive oil.

Nutrition Facts:

Per Serving; Calories 415; Fat 7.12g; Carbohydrates 72.4g; Protein 26.4g; Fiber 21.9g;

Lightning Source UK Ltd.
Milton Keynes UK
UKHW020747030621
384855UK00001B/135